Embracing Versatile Dieting:

Unlocking Health and Nutritional Success

By

James L. Hamilton

Disclaimer

The material presented in this book is for educational and informative purposes only. It is not meant as a replacement for professional medical advice, diagnosis, or treatment. Always seek the opinion of your physician or another competent health expert with any queries you may have about medical condition or food regimen.

Limit of Liability/Disclaimer of Warranty: The author and publisher have taken every effort to assure the correctness of the material presented. However, the material in this book is supplied "as is" without guarantee of any kind, either stated or implied, comprising but not restricted to the implicit guarantees of merchantability, fitness for a specific purpose, or non-infringement. The whole risk as to the quality, accuracy, and performance of the material is with the reader. In no circumstances will the author or publisher be responsible for any direct, consequential, incidental, special, punitive, or other damages whatsoever arising out of or in connection with the use of the book.

Table of contents

Embracing versatile dietin

Introduction

In today's fast-paced world, when fads come and go, one principle that has lasted the test of time is the necessity of a nutritious diet. However, the idea of a "healthy diet" has varied throughout the years, leaving many folks confused and overwhelmed. As we attempt to unleash our maximum potential in terms of health and nutrition, it's crucial to take a varied approach to dieting.

Welcome to the world of flexible dieting, where the emphasis is not on restrictive rules or rigorous meal plans but on the concepts of balance, flexibility, and uniqueness. This approach recognizes that each individual is unique, with varied dietary requirements and preferences. By choosing a varied diet, we open ourselves up to a world of options, enabling us to adjust our eating habits to fit our bodies and lives.

Gone are the days of one-size-fits-all diets that promise rapid solutions but frequently lead to disappointment.

Accepting varied diets implies accepting a mentality change — moving away from the concept of "good" and "bad" meals and instead adopting a more holistic approach on sustenance. It's about realizing that food is not only fuel for our bodies; it's a source of pleasure, cultural identity, and social connection.

In this journey towards health and nutritional success, we will cover the basic principles of flexible diets. We'll explore the power of mindful eating, which helps us to reconnect with our bodies and make conscious decisions. We'll dig into the practice of intuitive eating, where we learn to trust our internal signals and respect our hunger and fullness. Furthermore, we'll also discuss the advantages of adding a broad range of foods into our diets, enjoying the complex tapestry of tastes, textures, and nutrients accessible to us.

Moreover, we'll address the myth that flexible dieting is a free license to indulge in bad choices. On the contrary, it encourages us to prioritize nutrition while yet making space for occasional indulgences and enjoying the joys of life. By striking the correct balance, we can preserve our nutritional objectives while appreciating the pleasure of eating.

Throughout your trip, we'll rely on the latest scientific data, professional views, and practical suggestions to help you navigate the realm of flexible dieting effectively. Whether you're a seasoned health enthusiast or someone eager to begin on a new chapter of well-being, this investigation will equip you with the information and skills to unleash your full potential and achieve health and nutritional success.

So, let us begin on this revolutionary adventure together, as we plunge into the domain of flexible diets and uncover the secret to a better, more meaningful living. Prepare to embrace the power of balance, flexibility, and self-discovery as we start on this exciting trip towards optimum health and well-being.

Chapter 1

Embracing the realm of overeating and nutrition

In the area of overeating and nutrition, one strategy has been gaining pace and character for its inflexibility and effectiveness. Unlike restrictive diets that limit particular food orders or apply harsh restrictions, flexible overeating promotes variety and balance, making it a sustainable and enjoyable system to reach your health and nutritive objectives. In this post, we will bandy the notion of flexible overeating, its benefits, and how you might borrow it in your daily life.

1. Understanding protean Overeating
Defining varied Overeating: Learn what varied overeating comprises and how it varies from standard restrictive diets.

The Philosophy before different Dieting: Discover the ideas that uphold different overeating, similar as temperance, variety, and aware eating.

Breaking Free from Food Labels: Explore the notion of releasing oneself from labeling foods as" good" or" bad" and concentrating on general balance and temperance.

2. The Benefits of protean Overeating

Sustainable Weight Management: Understand how adaptable overeating supports long- term weight operation by avoiding the problems of inordinate and restrictive diets.

Improved Nutritional Intake: Explore how a diversified diet may guarantee you acquire a wide range of critical nutrients, vitamins, and minerals.

Enhanced Relationship with Food: Discover how varied overeating may make a healthy relationship with food, minimizing passions of guilt or privation.

3. Enforcing protean Overeating in Your Life
Structure a Balanced Plate: Learn about the factors of a different diet, including whole grains, spare flesh, fruits, vegetables, and healthy fats.

Meal Planning & Preparation: Get practical advice for introducing diversity into your reflections, including form ideas and mess-medication tactics.

Aware Eating and Portion operation: Understand the value of aware eating, harkening to your body's hunger and wholeness cues, and rehearsing portion operation.

4. Prostrating Challenges and risks
Dealing with jones and Emotional Eating: Discover ways to attack jones
and emotional eating within the environment of flexible overeating.

Dining Out & Social Events: Learn how to navigate caffs and social groups while keeping true to your adaptable salutary ideals.

Staying Motivated and harmonious: Find styles to maintain provocation and thickness on your varied overeating trip, including establishing realistic objects and measuring your success.

Embracing a varied overeating strategy may shift your relationship with food, enhance your nutritive input, and support long- term health and well- being. By embracing the generalities of temperance, diversity, and aware eating, you may establish a sustainable and enjoyable style of eating that supports your body while furnishing inflexibility and enjoyment. Flash back, flexible overeating is about embracing balance, not perfection, so start espousing these generalities into your everyday life and get the prices of a healthier, happier you.

Unlocking Health and Nutritional Success Key Strategies for a Vibrant Life

Achieving health and nutritive success is a continuance bid that needs trouble, understanding, and a comprehensive approach. In this post, we will cover essential tactics and ideas that can help open your path to optimal health and well- being.

From fueling your body with nutritional reflections to establishing aware actions, we will dig into concrete measures that will empower you to take charge of your health and experience the advantages of a full life.

1. Nourishing Your Body
The Power of Whole Foods: Understand the value of espousing a diet rich in whole, undressed foods that supply important nutrients and promote general health.

Balancing Macronutrients: Learn about the applicability of macronutrients(carbohydrates, proteins, and fats) and how to gain a balanced input for sustained energy and optimal functioning.

Prioritizing Micronutrients: Explore the significance of vitamins, minerals, and antioxidants in perfecting cellular health, adding impunity, and precluding nutrient deaths.

2. Aware Eating

Cultivating mindfulness: Discover the discipline of aware eating, which entails being present at the moment, savoring each mess, and paying attention to hunger and wholeness pointers.

Emotional Eating and Food Relationship: Learn how to describe emotional triggers and make ways to handle them successfully, developing a better relationship with food.

Portion operation and aware: Food Choices Understand the significance of portion operation and making aware food choices that match with your nutritive pretensions.

3. Hydration and Wellness:

The Significance of Hydration: Explore the multiple advantages of being hydrated, including improved digestion, greater cognitive performance, and healthier skin.

Optimal Water Intake: Learn how to determine and satisfy your unique hydration needs, taking into consideration parameters such as body weight, activity level, and environment.

Infusing Wellness with Hydration: Discover inventive methods to infuse your water with natural tastes, such as fruits and herbs, to enhance taste and raise your total fluid consumption.

4. Physical Activity and Exercise:
Finding Your Fitness Passion: Explore numerous forms of physical activities and training regimens to discover what matches your tastes and goals, assuring consistency and fun.

Establishing a Balanced Routine: Learn the benefits of implementing a balance of aerobic exercise, weight training, and flexibility exercises to increase overall fitness and well-being.

Making Movement a Lifestyle: Discover techniques to incorporate physical exercise into your everyday life, such as taking active breaks, using active transportation, or engaging in leisure activities.

5. Lifestyle Habits for Longevity:
Quality Sleep: Understand the critical importance of sleep in boosting physical and mental health, and discover techniques for enhancing sleep quality and developing a consistent sleep regimen.

Stress Management: Explore stress reduction approaches, including mindfulness, meditation, deep breathing exercises, and engaging in hobbies or activities that bring you joy.

Prioritizing Self-Care: Recognize the relevance of self-care activities that foster your mental, emotional, and physical well-being, and build a tailored self-care routine.

Unlocking health and nutritional success involves a complete strategy that incorporates fueling your body, practicing mindful eating, keeping hydrated, engaging in regular physical exercise, and emphasizing lifestyle choices that enhance longevity. By incorporating these tactics into your everyday life, you can take responsibility for your health, enjoy greater energy, and uncover a life of well-being and pleasure.

Remember, every tiny step matters, so start now and go on your road to a lively and healthy existence.

Achieving Balance: The Dynamic Duo of Diet and Exercise for Optimal Health

When it comes to obtaining optimal health and well-being, two important components play a critical role: nutrition and exercise.

Both parts are interwoven and operate synergistically to sustain a healthy body weight, boost overall fitness, and promote long-term health. In this post, we will cover the benefits of keeping a balanced diet and including regular exercise into your lifestyle. By knowing their distinct advantages and how they complement each other, you may unlock the potential of this powerful pair and reach your health and fitness objectives.

1. The Role of Diet:

Understanding Nutritional Needs: Learn about the fundamental macronutrients (carbohydrates, proteins, and fats) and micronutrients (vitamins and minerals) essential for optimal functioning and health.

Nourishing Your Body: Explore the benefits of adopting a balanced diet that includes whole, nutrient-dense foods, and learn the influence of adequate nutrition on energy levels, immunity, and general well-being.

Developing Healthy Eating Habits: Discover ways for introducing more fruits, vegetables, whole grains, lean proteins, and healthy fats into your diet, while reducing processed foods, sugar, and bad fats.

2. The Importance of Exercise:

Cardiovascular Health: Understand how regular aerobic activity, such as walking, jogging, or cycling, may strengthen your heart, improve circulation, and minimize the risk of cardiovascular illnesses.

Strength and Endurance: Explore the benefits of strength training activities to develop muscle, enhance bone density, and improve overall physical performance.

Mental & Emotional Well-being: Discover how exercise produces endorphins, decreases stress, raises mood, and promotes cognitive function, leading to enhanced mental and emotional well-being.

3. Synergistic Benefits of Diet and Exercise:

Weight Management: Learn how the combination of a good diet and regular exercise may help maintain a healthy body weight by establishing a calorie deficit, improving metabolism, and keeping lean muscle mass.

Energy and Stamina: Understand how adequate diet and regular physical activity synergistically lead to higher energy levels, greater endurance, and enhanced performance in daily tasks.

Disease Prevention: Explore the impact of nutrition and exercise in lowering the risk of chronic illnesses, such as obesity, type 2 diabetes, cardiovascular diseases, and some forms of cancer.

4. Strategies for Incorporating Diet and Exercise into Your Lifestyle:

Goal Setting: Learn how to create realistic objectives for both your food and exercise regimen, considering your present fitness level, preferences, and long-term desires.

Meal Planning & Prepping: Discover the benefits of meal planning and preparation to ensure a balanced diet, save time, and make better food choices.

Finding Enjoyable Exercise: Explore several sorts of physical activities, from sports to group fitness courses, to find what matches your interests and keeps you motivated.

Creating a pattern: Learn how to build a consistent pattern that involves regular exercise sessions and nutritious meals, making them a natural part of your everyday life.

5. Seeking Professional Guidance:
Consulting a Registered Dietitian: Understand the benefits of getting counsel from a registered dietitian to receive specialized nutrition recommendations and help in attaining your dietary objectives.

Engaging with a Fitness expert: Discover the benefits of working with a fitness expert, such as a personal trainer, to obtain individualized workout routines, appropriate form teaching, and continuing motivation.

Diet and exercise are vital components of a healthy lifestyle, functioning in harmony to support optimal health, weight control, and general well-being. By embracing a healthy diet rich in nutrients and combining regular physical activity into your routine, you may unlock the full potential of this powerful.

Optimal Health Diet: Nourishing Your Body for Lifelong Well-being

Adopting an ideal health diet is a major step towards boosting your general well-being, promoting lifespan, and minimizing the risk of chronic illnesses. By concentrating on nutrient-dense meals and mindful eating practices, you may fuel your body with the critical nutrients it needs to flourish. In this article, we will cover the essential concepts and components of an optimum health diet, allowing you to make educated choices and design a sustainable eating plan that supports your long-term health objectives.

1. Emphasize Nutrient-Dense Foods:
Whole Grains: Incorporate whole grains such as brown rice, quinoa, oats, and whole wheat bread, which are high in fiber, vitamins, and minerals.

Colorful Fruits and Vegetables: Include a variety of fruits and vegetables of different hues to provide a wide range of vitamins, minerals, antioxidants, and fiber.

Lean Proteins: Choose lean sources of protein such as skinless poultry, fish, lentils, tofu, and low-fat dairy products, which supply vital amino acids and improve muscle health.

Healthy Fats: Include sources of healthy fats like avocados, nuts, seeds, and olive oil, which deliver omega-3 fatty acids and improve heart health.

2. Balance Macronutrients:
Carbs: Prioritize complex carbs from whole grains, fruits, and vegetables, while minimizing the intake of processed grains and added sweets.

Proteins: Consume enough quantities of lean proteins, dispersing them throughout the day to assist muscle development, repair, and satiety.

Fats: Include sources of unsaturated fats such as avocados, nuts, seeds, and fatty fish, while reducing saturated and trans fats found in processed meals and fried goods.

3. Mindful Eating Habits:
Portion Control: Practice portion control by listening to your body's hunger and fullness cues, and prevent overeating by eating deliberately and carefully.

Mindful Meal Planning: Plan and prepare meals in advance to minimize depending on convenience foods, and consider combining meal preparing strategies to ensure healthful alternatives are easily available.

Mindful munching: Choose nutrient-dense snacks like fresh fruits, veggies with hummus, Greek yogurt, or almonds, and avoid mindless munching on processed and high-calorie items.

4. Hydration and Beverage Choices:
Water: Stay appropriately hydrated by drinking lots of water throughout the day, aiming for at least 8 glasses (64 ounces) or more depending on your activity level and climate.

Limit Sugary Drinks: Minimize or avoid sugary beverages including sodas, fruit juices, and energy drinks, as they are rich in added sugars and deliver empty calories.

Herbal Teas and Infused Water: Opt for herbal teas or infused water with natural tastes like lemon, cucumber, or mint to improve taste without additional sugars or artificial sweeteners.

5. Individualization and Moderation:
Bio Individuality: Recognize that ideal health diets may differ based on individual requirements, tastes, and any special dietary limitations or allergies you may have.

Moderation: Enjoy your favorite meals in moderation, exercising mindful pleasure while preserving overall balance and portion management.

Adopting an ideal health diet is a transforming journey that entails fueling your body with nutrient-dense foods, developing mindful eating habits, and embracing a balanced approach. By prioritizing whole grains, colorful fruits and vegetables, lean proteins, and healthy fats, you may fuel your body with the vital nutrients it needs for optimal performance and general well-being.

Unlocking health and nutritional success is a transforming path that allows individuals to take ownership of their well-being and make educated decisions about their food and lifestyle.

By recognizing the significance of balanced eating, combining regular exercise, and adopting healthy behaviors, individuals may experience a range of benefits, including higher energy levels, enhanced physical fitness, reduced risk of chronic illnesses, and overall well-being. It is vital to emphasize full, nutrient-dense meals, participate in regular physical activity, and create mindful eating habits. Additionally, obtaining professional help from registered dietitians and fitness professionals may give significant support and specific recommendations to enhance health and nutritional performance. Remember, little, persistent measures towards a healthy lifestyle can offer huge long-term advantages. By unlocking health and nutritional success, individuals may reach a greater quality of life, experience vitality, and thrive in all parts of their everyday lives.

Embracing a diversified diet is a powerful approach to fuel your body, promote your general health, and enjoy a broad range of flavors and culinary experiences. By ingesting a wide variety of nutrient-dense meals from different food categories, you may guarantee that your body obtains a balanced assortment of vitamins, minerals, and important elements. A diverse diet allows you to explore other cuisines, experiment with new ingredients, and find delight in the process of preparing and eating meals. Moreover, a diversified diet can help minimize food monotony, support good weight control, and lower the risk of nutrient shortages. Remember, a diverse diet is not about hard rules or limits but about appreciating the multitude of tastes and sustenance that nature delivers. So, let your taste sensations guide you as you start on a gastronomic trip that celebrates both health and fun.

Chapter 2

Metabolic response: maintaining energy balance

Metabolic response in the body involves a complex network of biochemical reactions and activities that occur to maintain energy balance and sustain cellular function. Here are some essential characteristics of metabolic reaction in the body:

Macronutrient Metabolism: The metabolic response includes the breakdown and use of macronutrients—carbohydrates, lipids, and proteins. Carbohydrates are turned into glucose, which is either utilized immediately for energy or stored as glycogen in the liver and muscles. Fats undergo lipolysis to release fatty acids for energy generation, whereas proteins are broken down into amino acids that may be used for numerous metabolic activities.

Energy generation: The metabolic response is largely focused on energy generation. Through a variety of interrelated mechanisms including glycolysis, the citric acid cycle (Krebs cycle), and oxidative phosphorylation, energy-rich molecules like ATP are created. ATP serves as the principal energy source for cellular functions, such as muscular contraction, neuronal signaling, and biosynthesis.

Hormonal Regulation: Hormones play a critical role in metabolic response and assist coordinate numerous metabolic processes. For example, insulin, produced by the pancreas, controls glucose metabolism by encouraging its absorption into cells and storage as glycogen. Glucagon, another pancreatic hormone, accelerates glycogen breakdown and enhances glucose release from the liver. Hormones including cortisol, growth hormone, and thyroid hormones can impact metabolism and energy balance.

Metabolic Rate: The metabolic response impacts the basal metabolic rate (BMR), which is the energy expenditure necessary to maintain fundamental body activities at rest.

BMR is affected by variables such as body composition, age, gender, and heredity. Higher muscle mass and physical activity levels normally boost BMR, whereas factors like age and certain medical problems might reduce it.

Thermogenesis: Metabolic response includes thermogenesis, the creation of heat by the organism. This mechanism helps control body temperature, especially in reaction to changes in the external environment. Thermogenesis may be stimulated by shivering, non-shivering thermogenesis (primarily in brown adipose tissue), and adaptive changes in blood flow and sweat production.

Nutrition Storage and Utilization: The metabolic response comprises nutrition storage and utilization to maintain energy balance. Excess glucose is stored as glycogen in the liver and muscles, which may be broken down and released as required.
Similarly, excess dietary fats are retained in adipose tissue as triglycerides for long-term energy storage. Proteins may also be employed as an energy source during extended fasting under specific physiological situations.

Metabolic Adaptations: The metabolic response displays flexibility to changing situations such as fasting, physical activity, and nutrition availability. During times of fasting, the body changes to other fuel sources, including stored fat and ketone bodies generated from fatty acids. Regular exercise may boost metabolic efficiency and produce beneficial adaptations, such as better insulin sensitivity and greater mitochondrial activity.

Understanding and improving metabolic response is critical for maintaining a healthy weight, controlling chronic conditions like diabetes and obesity, and fostering general well-being. It entails adopting a balanced diet, frequent physical exercise, and lifestyle choices that encourage efficient energy metabolism and metabolic flexibility. Consulting healthcare experts or licensed dietitians may give individualized counsel for those wishing to enhance their metabolic response.

Nutrient preservation and consumption

Nutrient preservation and intake play crucial roles in supporting a balanced diet and general well-being. Proper preservation procedures guarantee that the nutritional worth of foods is kept, while learning how to eat nutrients properly helps us to enjoy their advantages. Here are some essential steps to consider:

1. Importance of Nutrient Preservation:
Nutrient Retention: Proper preservation procedures help retain the vitamins, minerals, and other critical components in foods, ensuring they stay intact until consumption.

Extended Shelf Life: Effective preservation techniques improve the lifetime of perishable foods, decreasing waste and providing a consistent supply of nutrient-rich alternatives.

Food Safety: Preservation procedures, such as canning, pickling, and freezing, assist restrict the development of hazardous germs, assuring the safety of the food supply.

2. Preservation Methods:
Canning: This procedure includes sealing food in airtight containers and heating them to eradicate bacteria. It retains the nutritional content and increases the shelf life of fruits, vegetables, and even meats.

Freezing: Freezing foods at low temperatures slows down enzyme activity and microbiological development. Many fruits, vegetables, meats, and prepared meals may be properly preserved by freezing.

Drying/Dehydrating: Removing moisture from foods helps restrict the development of bacteria. Dehydrated fruits, vegetables, and herbs maintain their nutritious value and may be kept for a long time.

Pickling/Fermenting: Immersing foods in a brine or fermenting them with beneficial bacteria maintains their nutritious value while offering extra probiotic advantages.

3. Nutrient Consumption Strategies:

Balanced Diet: Consuming a well-balanced diet rich in fruits, vegetables, whole grains, lean meats, and healthy fats guarantees a broad variety of necessary nutrients.

Portion Control: Pay attention to portion proportions to prevent overeating and maintain a healthy weight. This strategy provides for a healthy distribution of nutrients throughout the day.

Cooking Techniques: Opt for healthy cooking techniques such as steaming, grilling, instead of deep-frying or boiling, since these help maintain the nutritious content of meals.

Food Combinations: Pairing certain meals might boost nutrient absorption. For example, having vitamin C-rich meals alongside iron-rich foods enhances iron absorption.

Avoid Over processing: Minimize the intake of overly processed foods that frequently lose key nutrients during manufacture. Fresh, whole foods are often more nutrient-dense.

4. Nutrient-Dense Foods:

Fruits and Vegetables: These are good sources of vitamins, minerals, fiber, and antioxidants. Aim for a diversity of colorful selections to receive a broad range of nutrients.

Whole Grains: Include whole grains like quinoa, brown rice, oats, and whole wheat, which give fiber, B-vitamins, and minerals.

Lean Proteins: Opt for lean sources of protein such as chicken, fish, tofu, beans, and lentils, which give critical amino acids for muscle repair and development.

Healthy Fats: Incorporate foods rich in healthy fats like avocados, nuts, seeds, and olive oil, which give omega-3 fatty acids and fat-soluble vitamins.

Dairy or Dairy substitutes: Consume low-fat dairy products or their substitutes such soy milk or almond milk for calcium, vitamin D, and protein. fruits, vegetables, and herbs maintain their nutritious value and may be kept for a long time.

Remember, nutrient preservation and consumption work hand in hand to guarantee you get the most out of your dietary choices. By applying correct preservation procedures and implementing wise consumption tactics, you may enjoy a well-rounded and nutrient-rich diet that adds to your overall health and vigor.

Nutritional cycling

Nutritional cycling, also known as nutrient cycling, refers to the ongoing transportation and modification of nutrients throughout the human system to support different physiological activities. The human body needs a broad spectrum of nutrients, including macronutrients (carbohydrates, proteins, and fats) and micronutrients (vitamins and minerals), to sustain optimum health and function. Nutritional cycling ensures that these important nutrients are absorbed, used, and recycled effectively.

Here are some major components of nutritional cycling in the body system:

Nutrient Absorption: The process of nutritional cycling starts with the absorption of nutrients from the food we ingest.
In the digestive tract, carbohydrates are broken down into glucose, proteins into amino acids, and fats into fatty acids. These nutrients are subsequently absorbed via the gut wall into the circulation.

Nutrient Distribution: Once absorbed, nutrients are carried through the bloodstream to various regions of the body where they are required. For instance, glucose is transferred to cells to give energy, amino acids are used for protein synthesis and tissue repair, and fatty acids are consumed for energy generation or stored as adipose tissue.

Nutrient Utilization: Within cells, nutrients undergo numerous metabolic processes to support critical tasks. Glucose is processed by cellular respiration to create adenosine triphosphate (ATP), the basic energy currency of the body.

Amino acids are integrated into proteins for development, maintenance, and repair of tissues. Fatty acids are broken down by beta-oxidation to create ATP or utilized as building blocks for cell membranes.

Nutrient Storage: Excess nutrients that are not immediately required for energy or cellular functions are saved for future use. Glucose is stored in the liver and muscles as glycogen, which may be swiftly turned back into glucose when energy needs grow. Fatty acids are stored as triglycerides in adipose tissue, providing a long-term energy reserve.

Nutrient Recycling: As the body continuously breaks down and rebuilds its tissues, nutrient recycling plays a key function. Amino acids produced during protein breakdown are utilized for the creation of new proteins. Similarly, minerals such as calcium and phosphorus are continually being deposited and taken from bones to preserve their strength and density.

Elimination of Waste: Alongside food cycling, the body also removes waste products created from metabolic activities. For example, carbon dioxide is created as a byproduct of cellular respiration and expelled via the lungs. Nitrogenous waste, such as urea, is expelled by the kidneys as urine.

Overall, nutritional cycling maintains a steady supply of nutrients for development, maintenance, and energy generation in the body.
It includes the effective absorption, distribution, usage, and recycling of nutrients, as well as the removal of waste products. A well-balanced diet, rich in a range of nutrients, is vital for supporting proper nutritional cycling and sustaining overall health.

Nutrient Planning

When it comes to weight reduction, a vital factor that frequently gets forgotten is nutrition planning. Proper nutritional consumption is vital for sustaining the body's functioning, boosting general health, and optimizing weight reduction efforts.

By concentrating on a well-balanced diet and integrating the correct nutrients, you may maximize your weight reduction journey and obtain sustained results. In this post, we will discuss the significance of nutrition planning and present practical recommendations to help you attain your weight reduction objectives.

1. Understand Your Calorie Needs:
Before getting into nutritional planning, it's necessary to estimate your daily calorie requirements. This may be done by determining your basal metabolic rate (BMR) utilizing internet calculators or speaking with a healthcare expert. Knowing your calorie needs will serve as a basis for designing a nutrient-rich food plan.

2. Prioritize Macronutrients:
Macronutrients, including carbs, proteins, and fats, play a significant role in weight reduction. Here's how to optimize each macronutrient:

Carbs: Choose complex carbs like whole grains, fruits, and vegetables over refined sugars and processed meals. They give sustained energy, fiber, and important vitamins and minerals.

Proteins: Incorporate lean sources of protein such as chicken, fish, tofu, lentils, and low-fat dairy products. Protein aids in developing and repairing tissues, improving satiety, and maintaining muscle mass during weight reduction.

Fats: Opt for healthy fats like avocados, nuts, seeds, and olive oil. These fats offer necessary fatty acids, enhance satiety, and assist food absorption. Limit saturated and trans fats present in fried and processed meals.

3.Micronutrients and Phytochemicals:
In addition to macronutrients, micronutrients and phytochemicals are equally vital for general health and weight reduction. Ensure your nutritional plan includes:

Vitamins and Minerals: Consume a mix of fruits, vegetables, whole grains, and lean proteins to acquire a wide spectrum of vitamins and minerals. These nutrients assist immunological function, energy generation, and cellular health.

Phytochemicals: Include a rainbow of colorful fruits and vegetables to benefit from the broad variety of phytochemicals they contain. These natural substances offer antioxidant effects, reduce inflammation, and contribute to general well-being.

4.Portion Control and Meal Frequency:
Maintaining optimal portion sizes and meal frequency is crucial for weight reduction. Consider the following tips:

Portion Control: Use smaller plates, bowls, and utensils to give the appearance of a bigger plate. Fill half your plate with veggies, one-quarter with lean protein, and one-quarter with healthy grains or starchy vegetables.

Meal Frequency: Aim for frequent, balanced meals throughout the day to regulate blood sugar levels and reduce overeating. Incorporate nutritious snacks between meals to keep hunger at bay and maintain energy levels.

5. Hydration:
Proper hydration is frequently forgotten yet is vital for weight reduction. Water assists with digestion,

lowers hunger, and boosts metabolism. Aim to drink an appropriate quantity of water every day and limit sugary drinks.

Nutrient planning is an essential element of a successful weight reduction journey. By concentrating on a well-balanced diet that contains macronutrients, micronutrients, and phytochemicals, you may optimize your body's functioning, support weight reduction efforts, and enhance overall health. Remember, it's crucial to work with a healthcare practitioner or registered dietitian to build a nutrition plan that meets your unique requirements and objectives. With a careful approach to nutrition planning, you may achieve long-term, sustainable weight reduction outcomes.

In conclusion, nutrition planning is a vital part of attaining effective and lasting weight reduction. By concentrating on a well-balanced diet that combines the correct macronutrients, micronutrients, and phytochemicals, you may optimize your body's processes, support your weight reduction efforts, and enhance your overall health.

Understanding your calorie demands, prioritizing macronutrients like carbs, proteins, and fats, and integrating lean sources of protein, complex carbohydrates, and healthy fats are critical elements in food planning for weight reduction. Additionally, providing an appropriate diet of vitamins, minerals, and phytochemicals via a broad variety of fruits, vegetables, whole grains, and lean meats is vital for general health and well-being.

Portion management, meal frequency, and hydration are equally critical parts of dietary planning. Practicing portion control, taking balanced meals at regular intervals, and being adequately hydrated will help regulate blood sugar levels, suppress cravings, and maintain healthy metabolism.

It's crucial to note that nutrition planning for weight reduction should be individualized and matched to individual requirements. Consulting with a healthcare expert or registered dietitian may give helpful insight and verify that your nutrition plan matches with your unique objectives and needs.

By taking a conscious and proactive approach to nutrition planning, you may boost your weight loss journey, obtain sustained outcomes, and create the basis for a healthy lifestyle overall. Remember that consistency and patience are crucial, and making incremental, lasting adjustments to your eating habits will bring the most substantial long-term advantages. With a well-planned food strategy, you can feed your body properly, maximize your weight reduction efforts, and begin on a road towards increased health and well-being.

Chapter 3

Healthy Eating: A Guide to Consuming Nutritious and Balanced Meals

Maintaining a healthy lifestyle starts with making deliberate decisions about what we consume. Adopting a healthy and balanced diet not only feeds our bodies with important nutrients but also helps avoid chronic illnesses, enhances energy levels, and promotes general well-being. In this thorough book, we will study the concepts of healthy eating and discover how to design a diet that is both enjoyable and nutritious.

Adopting a nutritious and balanced approach to eating is the cornerstone for a healthy lifestyle. By concentrating on eating full, nutrient-dense meals and maintaining a balanced intake of vital nutrients, we may enhance our general health and well-being.

With the practical strategies and meal ideas included in this book, you now have the skills to make educated decisions and prepare tasty, healthy meals that will support your path towards a better self. Remember, healthy eating is not about limitation but rather about adopting a sustainable and joyful manner of feeding your body. Start now and receive the advantages of a well-balanced diet for years to come.

The notion of nutritious and balanced meals is the cornerstone of a healthy lifestyle. Understanding the significance of fueling our bodies with the correct balance of nutrients may have a tremendous influence on our general well-being. In this tutorial, we will dig into the basics of healthy and balanced meals, studying the advantages they bring, the major components of such meals, and practical strategies for implementing them into our everyday lives.

Maintaining Weight and Promoting Better Digestive Health

Maintaining a healthy weight and fostering good gut health are key parts of overall well-being. By adopting mindful eating habits, choosing healthy food choices, and embracing lifestyle behaviors that assist digestion, you may reach a balanced weight and enhance your digestive function. In this tutorial, we will discuss practical techniques to help you manage weight and boost your gut health for a happier and better life.

Maintaining a healthy weight is a lifetime endeavor that needs a balanced approach to nutrition, exercise, and lifestyle decisions. While weight loss might be tough, it's crucial to concentrate on sustainable activities that improve overall well-being. Here are some crucial elements to remember while describing the maintenance of healthy weight reduction:

Set reasonable objectives: Start by defining attainable and feasible weight loss goals.
Aim for modest and steady improvement rather than quick weight reduction, since this is more sustainable in the long term.

Balanced diet: Adopting a balanced and nutritious diet is vital for healthy weight loss. Include a mix of fruits, vegetables, whole grains, lean meats, and healthy fats in your meals. Avoid fad diets or excessive limitations, since they are generally unsustainable and may deprive your body of important nutrients.

Portion control: Pay attention to portion proportions to prevent overeating. Use smaller dishes, bowls, and utensils to help manage your servings visually. Eating attentively, appreciating each meal, and listening to your body's hunger and fullness signals may help reduce overeating.

Regular physical exercise: Engage in regular physical activity to assist weight loss and general health. Aim for a mix of aerobic workouts, such as brisk walking, running, or cycling, together with strength training exercises to create lean muscle mass. Find things you like to make fitness a sustainable part of your routine.

Hydration: Stay appropriately hydrated by drinking lots of water throughout the day. Water may help suppress appetite and avoid overeating, since thirst is frequently mistaken for hunger. Replace sugary drinks with water or herbal teas to lower calorie consumption.

Sleep and stress management: Prioritize excellent sleep and handle stress properly. Lack of sleep may affect hormones linked to hunger and lead to weight gain. High stress levels might sometimes contribute to emotional eating or bad food choices. Engage in relaxation methods such as meditation, yoga, or deep breathing exercises to handle stress.

Behavior modification: Identify and address harmful eating behaviors or emotional triggers that lead to overeating. Seek help from a licensed dietitian or therapist who can aid with behavior modification strategies and give direction on establishing lasting lifestyle changes.

Accountability and support: Surround yourself with a support system of friends, family, or a weight loss group.
Sharing your objectives, efforts, and problems with others may give accountability and incentive. Additionally, try recording your food consumption and physical activity using apps or diaries to assess your progress.

Long-term mindset: Shift your emphasis from short-term weight reduction to long-term health and well-being. Embrace the notion of a healthy lifestyle rather than a transitory diet. Understand that weight fluctuations are natural and that maintaining a healthy weight is an ongoing endeavor.

Regular check-ins: Schedule regular check-ins with healthcare specialists to monitor your progress and get advice. They may make specific advice based on your individual requirements and help you remain on track.

Remember, keeping a healthy weight is not only about beauty but also about improving general health and quality of life. By taking a balanced strategy and implementing durable lifestyle modifications, you may achieve and maintain a healthy weight loss.

Sustainable practice in diet approach

Adopting a sustainable approach to eating is crucial to long-term success in maintaining a healthy weight and supporting overall well-being. Rather than following restrictive or fad diets, sustainable eating focuses on creating permanent improvements to your eating patterns and relationship with food. Here are few points to emphasize the relevance of sustainable practices in diet:

Balance and moderation: Sustainable eating promotes balance and moderation in dietary choices. Instead of fully eliminating particular food categories or engaging in severe limitations, strive for a well-rounded diet that incorporates a range of nutrients. This allows you freedom and fun while yet fueling your body.

Nutrient-dense foods: Prioritize nutrient-dense foods that offer a broad variety of critical elements, such as vitamins, minerals, fiber, and antioxidants. These include fruits, vegetables, entire grains, lean proteins, and healthy fats. By concentrating on nutrient-rich foods, you may fulfill your body's demands while limiting your calorie consumption.

Portion control: Paying attention to portion proportions is vital for sustainable eating. It's crucial to grasp the distinction between portion sizes and serving sizes, since they may sometimes vary. Using measuring cups, weighing scales, or visual clues may help you practice portion control and avoid overeating.

Mindful eating: Engage in mindful eating techniques, which entail being completely present and conscious of your food choices, eating patterns, and hunger signals. Slow down when eating, appreciate each mouthful, and heed to your body's cues of hunger and fullness. This helps you develop a standard connection with food and deletes emotional eating.

Gradual alterations: Instead of making radical changes overnight, try for gradual and sustained improvements to your diet. This permits your body and mind to adjust to new behaviors over time.
Start by integrating tiny, manageable adjustments, such as adding another serving of vegetables to your

meals or replacing sugary snacks for healthy choices.

Freedom and delight: Sustainable eating offers you freedom and enjoyment in your food choices. Allowing yourself to indulge sometimes in your favorite snacks or meals may help eliminate feelings of deprivation and build a healthy connection with food. It's about striking a balance between fueling your body and enjoying the meals you love.

Plan and prepare meals: Planning and preparing your meals in advance will help you make better choices throughout the week. Set aside some time each week to design a meal plan, compile a shopping list, and cook healthy meals and snacks. This lowers the dependence on processed or convenience meals, which are generally heavy in harmful fats, sugar, and salt.

Mindful supermarket shopping: Employ mindful purchasing groceries by selecting whole, unprocessed foods and reading food labels to make informed decisions. Prioritize fresh vegetables, lean proteins, healthy grains, and minimally processed products. Avoid highly processed foods that are heavy in chemicals, preservatives, and added sugars.

Hydration: Drinking a proper quantity of water is a crucial aspect of a sustainable diet. It helps maintain appropriate physical processes, assists digestion, and may avoid overeating by keeping you hydrated. Make it a habit to carry a water bottle with you and sip on water throughout the day.

Seek assistance: Building a support system may substantially aid sustainable eating. Surround yourself with like-minded persons who are likewise focused on good practices. Consider taking a cooking class, a nutrition support group, or obtaining help from a certified dietitian who can give tailored advice and support.

By maintaining a sustainable approach to nutrition, you may create healthy eating habits that will support your long-term well-being.
Remember that everyone's path is unique, so it's vital to determine what works best for you and make

changes at a speed that is sustainable for your lifestyle.

Fostering good eating habits is critical for our general well-being and plays a significant part in sustaining a healthy lifestyle. By selecting a balanced and healthy diet, we give our bodies the vital nutrients, energy, and building blocks required for optimum functioning.
You may build good eating habits that promote optimum health, assist weight control, and contribute to your general well-being. Remember, tiny adjustments over time may lead to huge benefits, so enjoy the path towards a healthy self.

In conclusion, adopting a sustainable practice in a diet strategy is vital for long-term success in sustaining a healthy lifestyle. By focusing on balance, moderation, and mindful eating, you may build a healthy connection with food and make decisions that promote your overall well-being.

Sustainable eating entails ingesting a variety of nutrient-dense meals, exercising portion management, and being conscious of your body's hunger and fullness signals. It also highlights the significance of eating complete, minimally processed meals, reducing added sweets and harmful fats, and utilizing local and seasonal fruit. Planning and preparing meals, keeping hydrated, and allowing for flexibility and pleasure in your food choices are all critical components of sustainable eating. Remember, sustainable practices are not about tight restrictions or fast cures but about adopting incremental, lasting adjustments that enhance health and harmony with the environment. By accepting these ideas, you may begin on a sustainable eating path that feeds both your health and the world.

Stabilization of healthy diet

Stabilizing a healthy diet is vital for long-term success in sustaining a nutritious and balanced eating routine. While establishing a healthy diet is crucial, it is necessary to maintain it over time.

Here are some crucial elements to consider while striving to stabilize a healthy diet:

Consistency is key: Consistency is the cornerstone of a consistent healthy diet. Stick to your selected eating pattern and make it a part of your everyday habit. Avoid short-term or crash diets that are difficult to keep and instead concentrate on establishing persistent adjustments to your eating habits.

Set reasonable and attainable objectives: Develop achievable and achievable objectives that match with your lifestyle, tastes, and nutritional requirements. Avoid setting stringent or too ambitious objectives that may lead to dissatisfaction and make it tougher to follow the diet in the long term. Gradual improvement is more sustainable and simpler to maintain.

Plan your meals: Plan your meals in advance to ensure you have healthful selections readily accessible. Meal planning helps you make better choices, saves time, and decreases the dependence on harmful convenience foods.

Set aside time each week to establish a meal plan, compile a shopping list, and prepare items in advance.

Stock up on healthy food options: Keep your pantry, refrigerator, and freezer stocked with a range of nutritious food choices. Include fruits, vegetables, whole grains, lean meats, and healthy fats on your grocery list. Having nutritious foods readily accessible makes it simpler to make good choices when hunger hits.

Practice portion control: Pay attention to portion proportions to prevent overeating. Use measuring cups, kitchen scales, or visual indicators to ensure you're ingesting adequate quantities. Practice mindful eating by enjoying each mouthful, eating deliberately, and listening to your body's hunger and fullness cues.

Keep Nutritional snacks on hand: Prepare as well as portion out nutritional treats in advance. conclude for choices like fresh fruits, veggies with hummus, Greek yogurt, almonds, or manual energy snacks. Having these snacks readily accessible will help you avoid reaching for dangerous options when anger arises between reflections.

Stay focused: Proper hydration is vital for sustaining a balanced diet. Drink an applicable volume of water throughout the day. Carry a water bottle with you as a memorial to remain doused . Water helps control hunger, assists digestion, and promotes general health.

Practice temperance, not privation:. Allow yourself to enjoy your favorite reflections in temperance. Depriving oneself of pleasures might lead to feelings of constraint and eventually end in binge- eating or slipping off track. Exercise conscious indulgence and relish little servings of your favorite delectables occasionally.

Seek help and responsibility: Partake your healthy eating objects with a probative friend, family member, or join a community or support group. Having someone to bandy your sweats, problems, and accomplishments with may give incitement and responsibility.

Be flexible and acclimatize: Life is full of unanticipated circumstances, social occasions, and fests that may test your healthy eating habits.
It's pivotal to be adaptable and acclimate to changing conditions without feeling shamefaced.

Allow yourself to appreciate exceptional moments while keeping a balanced station overall.

Flash back: Sustaining a healthy diet is a constant process that involves fidelity, tolerance, and tone-compassion. Embrace the trip, concentrate on progress rather than perfection, and appreciate the good advancements you make along the way. With time and trouble, a healthy diet will become a natural and sustainable part of your life.

How to boost your healthy diet

Perfecting your healthy diet is a precious exertion that may have a great influence on your entire well-being. By making modest and patient variations to your eating habits, you may increase the nutritive content of your diet. Then are some pivotal rudiments to consider while seeking to enhance your healthy diet

Assess your eating habits: Begin by examining the present salutary habits and changing areas for enhancement. Take note of any dangerous trends, similar as inordinate consumption of reused reflections, sticky potables, or inadequate input of fruits and vegetables.

Increase fruit and vegetable input: Aim to incorporate a variety of fruits and veggies in your regular reflections. They're rich with important vitamins, minerals, and fiber. trial with colorful kinds, colors, and medications to make them more seductive and enjoyable.

Choose whole grain

Conclude for whole grain druther like whole wheat, brown rice, quinoa, and oats rather than reused grains. Whole grains are richer in fiber and deliver further nutrients, enabling better digestion and long- continuing energy.

Prioritize spare proteins: Incorporate spare sources of protein into your reflections, similar as skinless funk, fish, lentils, tofu, and low- fat dairy products. Protein is demanded for muscle development, form, and malnutrition.

Reduce added sugars: Cut down on reflections and drinks that contain added sugars, similar as tonics, sweets, sticky cereals, and ignited goods. conclude for naturally candied products like fresh fruits or thin druthers
.

Minimize reused foods: Limit your consumption of reused foods rich in added sugars, dangerous fats, and swab.

These include fast food,pre-packaged snacks, and frozen reflections. rather, go for complete, undressed reflections wherever doable.

Include able-bodied fats: Incorporate sources of healthy fats into your diet, similar as avocados, nuts, seeds, and olive oil painting. These fats give critical nutrients and may ameliorate heart health.

Hydrate with water: Make water your main libation option. Avoid sticky drinks and circumscribe the operation of alcohol. Staying adequately doused helps save overall health and assists with digestion.

Practice aware eating: Pay attention to your body's hunger and wholeness signals. Eat gently and delight each nibble, concentrating on the tastes and textures of your mess. aware eating may help you better descry whether you're actually empty or quenched.

Seek expert counsel: Consider meeting with a certified dietitian or nutritionist for specific advice and guidance.

They may examine your individual salutary conditions, make advice, and make a substantiated mess plan to help you ameliorate your healthy eating habits.

Strategy and prepare reflections: Set away time each week to plan and prepare your reflections. This lets you have nutritional choices fluently accessible, barring the temptation to elect for less healthy druthers while you are busy or on the move.

Embrace modest changes: Flashback that changing your healthy diet constitutes a nonstop process. Start by making bitsy, attainable variations to your salutary habits and make upon them over time. This system raises the chance of long- term success.

Be nice to yourself with a nutritional diet: Focus on progress rather than perfection and enjoy each step you take towards a healthy living.

Perfecting your healthy diet is a continual and ongoing exertion. By enforcing these tactics and precipitously making better choices, you may enhance your nutritive input and promote your overall well- being.

Chapter 4

How to integrate exercise and physical activity

Incorporating fitness and physical activity into your routine may be a gratifying and joyful experience. Here are some practical strategies to help you make physical exercise a regular part of your life:

Set reasonable objectives: Start by creating reasonable and attainable objectives. Whether it's aiming for a particular number of weekly exercises or raising your daily step count, creating precise objectives may help you remain focused and motivated.

Locate Activities You appreciate: Explore numerous sorts of physical activities to locate ones that you actually appreciate.

It may be dancing, swimming, cycling, hiking, playing a sport, or even attending a group fitness class. When you discover hobbies that you look forward to, it becomes simpler to remain with them.

Schedule Your Workouts: Treat exercise like any other essential appointment by arranging it into your schedule. Block out particular hours during the week devoted to physical exercise. Consistency is crucial, so try to make it a habit to exercise at the same time each day or on specified days of the week.

Start gently and Gradually Increase Intensity: If you're new to exercising, it's crucial to start gently and gradually increase the intensity and length of your exercises. This helps avoid injuries and enables your body to adjust to the demands of exercise. You may begin with shorter sessions and low-impact exercises, then gradually build up to more strenuous routines.

Make It a Social exercise: Exercising with a friend, family member, or a workout group may make physical exercise more fun and help you remain motivated.

You may organize regular gym sessions together, go for walks or runs with a partner, or join fitness programs or sports teams where you can meet like-minded others.

Incorporate Physical Activity Into Daily Life: Look for chances to be active throughout the day. Take the stairs instead of the elevator, walk or cycle to work if feasible, park your vehicle further away from your destination to get in some additional steps, or take active breaks during sedentary times (e.g., stretching, brief walks).

Use Technology and applications: Utilize technology and fitness applications to measure your progress, create objectives, and remain inspired. There are various applications available that may help you count your steps, document your activities, give training programs, or even deliver virtual lessons and assistance.

Mix It Up: To keep things interesting, diversify your exercises and hobbies.

Try varied workouts, explore outdoor activities in nature, or join fitness challenges to keep yourself involved and
motivated. Variety not only eliminates boredom but also helps train various muscle groups and enhances overall fitness.

Be Mindful of Safety: Prioritize your safety while physical exercise. Warm up before each exercise, wear suitable clothes and footwear, remain hydrated, and listen to your body. If you encounter any pain or discomfort, alter or reduce your activities appropriately, and seek expert guidance if required.

Celebrate Your Achievements: Acknowledge and celebrate your successes along the road. Whether it's completing a fitness milestone, boosting your endurance, or just sticking to your training regimen, reward yourself to remain motivated and reinforce healthy behaviors.

Remember, consistency is crucial when it comes to implementing exercise and physical activity into your routine. Start small, pick things you love, and gradually build up your fitness level.

With time, regular physical exercise will become a natural and pleasurable aspect of your existence.

How to maintain sustained fitness of health

Maintaining sustained fitness and health is vital for long-term well-being. Here are some ways to help you build and maintain a sustainable approach to your fitness and health:

Set reasonable objectives: Start by defining reasonable and attainable objectives that correspond with your lifestyle, preferences, and talents. Avoid establishing too ambitious or limiting objectives that may lead to fatigue or dissatisfaction. Focus on creating steady, sustainable adjustments that you can maintain over the long run.

Prioritize Consistency: Consistency is crucial to sustaining fitness and health. Create a regular fitness plan that incorporates things you love and can realistically fit into your schedule. Aim for consistency rather than intensity.

Even shorter exercises or physical activities done regularly might have a favorable influence on your overall fitness level.

Find Activities You Enjoy: Engage in physical activities that you find fun and gratifying. This might include engaging in a sport, dancing, hiking, swimming, cycling, or attending fitness courses. When you appreciate what you're doing, you're more likely to remain with it over time.

Mix Up Your program: Avoid becoming bored or plateauing by introducing variation into your training program. Explore various sorts of activities, try new courses or sports, or freshen up your training surroundings. Adding variation not only keeps things interesting but also pushes various muscle groups and avoids overuse issues.

Listen to Your Body: Pay attention to your body's cues and alter your training regimen appropriately. Rest and recuperate as required, and avoid pushing through discomfort or exhaustion that may lead to damage.

Remember, sustaining fitness includes taking care of your body and striking a balance between pushing yourself and allowing for healthy recuperation.

Practice thoughtful Eating: Adopt a thoughtful attitude to eating by listening to your body's hunger and fullness signals. Focus on having a balanced diet that includes complete, unprocessed foods and proper portion proportions. Avoid restrictive diets or severe eating behaviors that are not sustainable in the long term.

Stay Hydrated: Hydration is crucial for overall health and excellent physical performance. Drink water throughout the day to maintain hydration levels, particularly during activity or while in hot conditions. The actual quantity of water required varies based on variables such as activity intensity, climate, and individual demands.

Restorative Sleep: Prioritize great sleep as part of your overall health and fitness program. Aim for 7–9 hours of unbroken sleep each night. Create a peaceful nighttime ritual, build a sleep-friendly atmosphere, and follow excellent mattress hygiene behaviors.

Manage Stress: Chronic stress may significantly affect your fitness and general health. Find healthy strategies to handle stress, such as practicing relaxation techniques, participating in hobbies or activities you like, finding social support, and adding stress-reducing practices like meditation or yoga into your routine.

Frequent Health Check-ups: Schedule frequent check-ups with healthcare specialists to monitor your general health and well-being. These check-ups may help detect any possible difficulties early on and allow for appropriate treatments or modifications to your exercise and health program.

Remember, sustained fitness and health are about developing a lifestyle that promotes your well-being over the long run. It's crucial to establish balance, listen to your body, and make decisions that are fun and sustainable for you individually.

How to keep routine to burn calories and enhance metabolism

Maintaining a program to burn calories and raise metabolism needs a mix of regular physical exercise, good eating habits, and lifestyle choices. Here are some ways to help you keep such a routine:

Engage in Regular Exercise: Incorporate a combination of aerobic activities, strength training, and high-intensity interval training, or HIIT, into your fitness program. Aim for at least 150 minutes of moderate-intensity aerobic activity or 75 minutes of vigorous-intensity aerobic activity per week, combined with strength training activities at least twice a week. Consistency is crucial, so choose things you like and make them a regular part of your calendar.

Strength Training: Include strength training activities to increase and maintain muscle mass. Muscle is more metabolically active than fat, therefore having more muscle may improve your resting metabolic rate.

Incorporate exercises that target key muscular groups, such as squats, lunges, deadlifts, push-ups, and pull-ups.

High-Intensity Interval Training (HIIT): Integrate HIIT exercises into your program. HIIT comprises short bursts of intensive activity followed by shorter recuperation intervals. This sort of exercise has been demonstrated to enhance calorie burn and raise metabolism long after the session is over. Examples of HIIT activities include sprints, burpees, jump squats, or cycling at maximum effort for brief periods.

Stay Active Throughout the Day: Look for chances to be active in your everyday life. Take brief pauses to stretch or go for a quick walk, utilize the stairs instead of elevators, or explore standing workstations. These little actions may assist raise calorie expenditure and keep your metabolism active throughout the day.

Eat a Balanced Diet: Focus on a well-balanced diet that contains lean meats, whole grains, fruits, vegetables, and healthy fats.

Protein has a larger thermal impact, meaning it needs more energy to digest, which might temporarily raise metabolism. Fiber-rich diets can lead to increased calorie expenditure during digestion. Avoid crash diets or very low-calorie diets, since they might slow down your metabolism and contribute to muscle loss.

Stay Hydrated: Drink enough water throughout the day to promote optimal metabolism and general health. Water is needed for numerous metabolic functions, and even minor dehydration might severely impair your metabolism. Stay hydrated by consuming water often, and try substituting sugary beverages or sodas with water.

Get Sufficient Sleep: Prioritize quality sleep as lack of sleep might alter your metabolism. Poor sleep may disrupt hormone control, increase appetite, and lead to desires for bad eating choices. Establish a consistent sleep regimen, establish a sleep-friendly atmosphere, and practice soothing methods for improving the quality of your sleep.

Manage Stress: Chronic stress may impair your metabolism and lead to weight gain.

Find healthy strategies to handle stress, such as exercise, meditation, deep breathing, or participating in activities you like. Prioritize self-care and seek assistance when required to help manage stress levels successfully.

Monitor and alter: Regularly monitor your progress and alter your program as required. Monitor your calorie intake and expenditure, maintain a diet and activity record, or employ fitness apps to help you remain on track. Assess your progress, make any modifications to your program, and establish new objectives to continue pushing yourself.

Remember, keeping a program to burn calories and enhance metabolism is a long-term commitment. Consistency, perseverance, and adopting sustainable lifestyle choices are crucial to reaching and sustaining your desired outcomes. It's vital to listen to your body, seek expert assistance when required, and make decisions that match with your specific requirements and preferences.

Importance of keeping routine to burn calories and enhance metabolism.

Maintaining a routine is vital for burning calories and improving metabolism. Here are some fundamental reasons why it is crucial to stay to a regular routine:

Consistency in Physical Activity: Regular exercise and physical activity have a key part in burning calories and increasing metabolism. When you keep a routine, you build a habit of participating in regular exercise, whether it's cardio, strength training, or any other sort of physical activity. Consistency helps your body to adapt to the demands of exercise and enhance calorie burning and metabolic processes.

Sustained Caloric Expenditure: Burning calories takes constant effort over time. By keeping to a program, you guarantee that you're continuously participating in activities that boost your heart rate and increase energy expenditure. This prolonged caloric expenditure helps produce a calorie deficit, which is critical for weight reduction and control.

Muscle Development: Regular exercise not only burns calories throughout the activity but also aids in creating lean muscle mass. By keeping a regimen that combines strength training activities, you may improve your muscle mass, which in turn boosts your basal metabolic rate (BMR), leading to more calories expended throughout the day.

Regulation of Hormones: Consistency in exercising and keeping a routine may assist manage hormones associated with metabolism and hunger control. Physical exercise helps regulate hormones such as insulin, cortisol, leptin, and ghrelin, which play a critical role in energy control, fat accumulation, and hunger signals.

When these hormones are appropriately balanced, your body can effectively use calories, store less fat, and maintain a healthy metabolic rate.

Metabolic Adaptation: Our bodies are adaptive, and they adjust to our regular routines. When you continue a constant schedule of exercise and physical activity, your body gets more efficient at consuming energy and boosts its metabolic rate to match the demands of your routine.

This metabolic adaptation helps you burn calories more effectively and efficiently.

Long-Term Weight control: Establishing a regimen is vital for long-term weight control. Sustainable weight reduction and maintenance need regular practices rather than short-term efforts. By adding regular exercise and establishing a schedule, you develop a lifestyle that supports your weight control objectives by consistently burning calories and keeping your metabolism active.

Remember, although establishing a schedule is vital, it's equally necessary to listen to your body and avoid overtraining or pushing yourself too hard. It's essential to speak with a healthcare practitioner or a trained fitness expert to design a customized plan that meets your requirements and skills.

Increasing metabolism: healthy weight and promoting appropriate energy levels

Increasing metabolism is vital for maintaining a healthy weight, fostering adequate energy levels, and supporting general well-being. Here are some crucial aspects to consider when it comes to improving metabolism:

Focus on Regular Physical Activity: Engaging in regular exercise and physical activity is one of the most effective strategies to enhance metabolism. Incorporate a mix of aerobic activities, weight training, and high-intensity interval training (HIIT) to increase calorie burn during and after your workouts.

Develop strong Muscle Mass: Strength training activities in your program helps grow and maintain lean muscle mass, which improves your basal metabolic rate (BMR). Aim for a well-rounded fitness regimen that targets all main muscle groups.

Prioritize Protein Intake: Protein plays a key function in metabolism. It needs more energy to digest compared to fats or carbs, resulting in a transient rise in calorie expenditure.

Additionally, taking appropriate protein stimulates muscle development and repair, further boosting your metabolism. Include lean sources of protein such as chicken, fish, tofu, and lentils in your meals.

Don't Skip Meals: Irregular or insufficient calorie intake might contribute to a sluggish metabolism. Make sure to have balanced meals throughout the day and avoid lengthy periods of fasting. Fuel your body with a balance of nutrients from entire meals, including complex carbs, lean proteins, healthy fats, and fiber.

Stay Hydrated: Drinking adequate water is vital for maintaining a healthy metabolism. Water is involved in several metabolic processes, including the breakdown of carbohydrates and lipids. Aim to drink a suitable quantity of water throughout the day to maintain proper hydration and metabolism.

Get Sufficient Sleep: Lack of sleep may disturb hormonal balance and significantly affect metabolism. Aim for 7-9 hours of excellent sleep each night to promote general health, hormone control, and optimum metabolic function.

Remember that everyone's metabolism is unique, and variables such as genetics, age, and body composition may impact its pace. Focus on establishing a healthy lifestyle that involves regular exercise, a balanced diet, and appropriate relaxation to promote a healthy metabolism and general well-being.

Chapter 5

Lifestyle adjustments in diet: Implementing permanent modifications to your everyday habits and routine

Lifestyle adjustments in diet relate to improvements made to one's eating habits and choices in order to promote general health and well-being. These modifications may have a substantial influence on several parts of life, including physical health, emotional well-being, energy levels, and illness prevention. Here are some theories for distinct lifestyle changes in diet:

Reducing processed foods: Processed foods are generally heavy in harmful fats, added sugars, and artificial additives. By lowering their consumption, consumers may minimize their intake of empty calories, salt, and preservatives, and instead choose for full, unprocessed meals like vegetables, fruits, grains that are whole, and lean meats.

Incorporating more fruits and veggies: Fruits and vegetables are rich with critical vitamins, minerals, and fiber. By integrating a variety of colorful produce in your diet, you supply your body with vital nutrients that promote general health, stimulate the immune system, and minimize the risk of chronic illnesses.

Increasing water intake: Proper hydration is necessary for healthy biological functioning, including digestion, circulation, and temperature control. By consuming a proper quantity of water throughout the day, people may increase their energy levels, promote good skin, assist in weight control, and boost general well-being.

Portion management: Practicing portion control requires being careful of the amount of food ingested during meals. By listening to your body's hunger and fullness signals and adjusting portion sizes, you may prevent overeating, maintain a healthy weight, and avoid needless calorie consumption.

Mindful eating: Mindful eating is the discipline of paying attention to the sensory experiences and bodily feelings when ingesting food.

By slowing down, enjoying each mouthful, and being mindful of hunger and fullness signals, people may build a healthy connection with food, optimize digestion, and reduce overeating.

Including lean protein sources: Lean protein, such as chicken, fish, tofu, lentils, and low-fat dairy products, is important for muscle building, tissue repair, and hormone synthesis. Incorporating these protein sources into your diet will help you feel satisfied for longer, maintain a healthy body composition, and boost overall strength and vigor.

Limiting added sugars: Excessive intake of added sugars, frequently found in sugary drinks, processed snacks, and desserts, may lead to weight gain, diabetes, and other health concerns. By lowering your consumption of added sugars and choosing for natural sweeteners like fruits or stevia, you may minimize the risk of chronic illnesses and stabilize energy levels.

Choosing healthy fats: Not all fats are created equal. Opting for healthy fats like avocados, almonds, seeds, and olive oil instead of saturated and trans fats may support heart health, improve cognitive function, and help in nutritional absorption.

Planning and preparing meals: Planning and preparing meals in advance provides for better food choices and portion management. By keeping nutritious meals easily accessible, you are less likely to depend on harmful convenience foods or give in to impulsive, less healthy selections.

Regular physical exercise: While not directly connected to diet, regular physical activity complements a healthy eating plan by supporting weight control, lowering the risk of chronic illnesses, increasing mood, and enhancing general well-being. Incorporating exercise into your lifestyle might have a synergistic impact with dietary adjustments.

Remember, adopting lifestyle changes in nutrition is a long process, and it's crucial to work with a healthcare practitioner or registered dietitian to ensure these changes correspond with your individual health requirements and objectives.

Here are several take-up possibilities in upgrading your lifestyle adjustments

Reduce single-use plastic: Carry a reusable water bottle, coffee cup, and shopping bags to decrease the usage of throwaway products.
Possible
Eat a plant-based diet: Incorporate more fruits, vegetables, legumes, and whole grains into your meals while minimizing the intake of animal products. This may minimize your carbon impact and encourage healthy eating habits.

Use public transportation or carpool: Opt for public transit, bicycling, or walking whenever to decrease carbon emissions. If you need to utilize a vehicle, try carpooling with coworkers or friends to split the commute.

Conserve energy at home: Turn off lights and unplug electrical gadgets when not in use. Use energy-efficient products, such as LED light bulbs and smart power strips, to limit electricity use.

Reduce water usage: Take shorter showers, mend leaking taps, and collect rainwater for outdoor plants. Conserving water helps protect this unique resource.

Shop locally and sustainably: Support local farmers' markets and companies that promote sustainable and eco-friendly activities. Choose items with minimum packaging and search for organic or fair-trade choices.

Embrace thrift shopping: Instead of constantly purchasing new clothing, visit thrift shops or online platforms for old stuff. This eliminates waste and fosters a circular economy.

Minimize food waste: Plan meals in advance, keep leftovers appropriately, and compost organic waste. Being conscious of what you eat helps decrease food waste and its accompanying environmental effect.

Practice conscious consumerism: Before making a purchase, ask yourself whether you genuinely need the item and consider its sustainability. Invest in quality, robust items that will last longer and lessen the need for replacements.

Connect with nature: Spend time outside, whether it's gardening, hiking, or just taking a stroll in the park. Developing a stronger connection with nature creates respect and inspires you to safeguard the environment.

Reduce your carbon footprint: Use energy-efficient transportation choices, such as electric automobiles or hybrid cars, if practical. Offset your carbon emissions by supporting programs that promote renewable energy or reforestation.

Embrace minimalism: Declutter your living area and practice mindful living. Focus on experiences rather than material stuff, resulting in less waste and a simpler, more sustainable existence.

Engage in community initiatives: Participate in local environmental efforts, such as clean-up drives or community gardens. Collaborating with others multiplies your effect and generates a feeling of shared responsibility.

Educate yourself and others: Stay knowledgeable about environmental concerns and share your knowledge with friends and family. Encourage dialogues and encourage sustainable behaviors in your social groups.

Prioritize self-care: Engage in activities that relieve stress and increase well-being. Taking care of oneself helps you to maintain a sustainable lifestyle and motivate others to do the same.

Remember, making durable changes is a journey, and progress is more essential than perfection. Start with modest steps, gradually adding these habits into your daily routine, and celebrate each milestone along the way.

Here are some essential reasons why a diet should be a lifetime and not a weekly meal

A diet should be a lifestyle and not simply a weekly meal for numerous fundamental reasons:

Long-term sustainability: A diet that is handled as a lifestyle fosters sustainable and consistent behaviors. It emphasizes on establishing lasting adjustments to your eating habits and entire lifestyle rather than depending on short-term remedies. A weekly meal, on the other hand, is confined to a set time range and may not deliver permanent effects.

Health advantages: Adopting a nutritious diet as a habit may lead to several health benefits. It helps you to build balanced eating habits that offer important nutrients, encourage weight control, minimize the risk of chronic illnesses like heart disease and diabetes, and increase general well-being. A weekly meal, on the contrary, may not emphasize these long-term health objectives.

Thinking change: Embracing a diet as a lifestyle entails a thinking shift towards making better choices regularly. It encourages you to build a healthy connection with food, concentrating on nutrition and general wellbeing. A weekly meal may develop a transitory mentality focused on following a particular plan rather than adopting a comprehensive approach to eating.

Flexibility and adaptability: A diet as a lifestyle provides for flexibility and adaptation to varied contexts and life events. It helps you to make better choices in varied circumstances, such as social events, vacations, or holidays, without feeling constrained. A weekly menu may not give the same degree of flexibility and might lead to emotions of deprivation or guilt when straying from the plan.

Habit development: When a diet becomes a lifestyle, it facilitates the establishment of permanent habits. Consistently maintaining a healthy eating pattern over time helps consolidate these habits into your everyday routine. This makes it simpler to maintain a balanced diet in the long term, while a weekly menu may not give the same potential for habit building.

Overall well-being: A diet that becomes a lifestyle goes beyond simply the food you consume. It covers other lifestyle aspects including regular physical exercise, stress management, and enough sleep, all of which contribute to overall well-being. A weekly menu may not address these extra issues, perhaps overlooking crucial components of a healthy lifestyle.

In conclusion, accepting a diet as a lifestyle rather than a weekly menu provides various advantages in terms of sustainability, health benefits, attitude change, flexibility, habit development, and general well-being. It supports long-term success in developing and sustaining a healthy lifestyle, rather than focusing on short-term remedies.

How can I maintain a healthy diet and eat less?

Maintaining a nutritious diet and reducing portion sizes might be tough, but with some practical measures, it is attainable.

Here are some suggestions to help you maintain a balanced diet and less consumption:

Portion control: Be cautious of portion sizes by using smaller dishes and bowls. Fill half of your plate with veggies, one-quarter with lean protein, and one-quarter with healthy grains or starchy vegetables. This strategy helps you have a balanced meal while managing calorie consumption.

Plan and prepare your meals: Plan your meals and snacks in advance to prevent impulsive or unhealthy food choices. Preparing meals at home enables you to have control over ingredients and portion amounts. Pack your lunch and snacks for work or activities to avoid depending on convenience meals.

Include protein and fiber-rich food items: these nutrients assist generate satiety and keep you feeling fuller for longer. Incorporate lean sources of protein like chicken, fish, beans, and tofu into your meals. Include high-fiber meals like whole grains, fruits, vegetables, and legumes to provide bulk and assist digestion.

Stay hydrated: Sometimes we confuse thirst for hunger. Drink water throughout the day to keep hydrated and to discern between actual hunger and thirst. Water may also assist minimize overeating during meals.

Limit processed and sugary foods: Processed foods generally have extra sugars, harmful fats, and excess salt. Minimize your consumption of sugary snacks, drinks, packaged snacks, and fast meals. Opt for full, natural meals including vegetables, fruits, whole grains, lean meats, and healthy fats.

Be careful of liquid calories: Beverages including sugary sodas, fruit juices, energy drinks, and alcoholic beverages may contribute to excess calorie consumption. Choose water, herbal tea, or unsweetened drinks as your major drink options.

Practice portion awareness: Learn to identify proper portion sizes. Use measuring cups, a food scale, or visual clues to understand optimum serving quantities. This will assist you avoid eating greater quantities than required.

Identify emotional eating triggers: Emotional eating may lead to overeating or selecting unhealthy meals. Identify your triggers, such as tension, boredom, or grief, and discover alternate coping methods like exercise, meditation, or indulging in a hobby.

Seek help and accountability: Consider enlisting the assistance of a friend, family member, or joining a support group or online community focused on healthy eating. Sharing your experience with others may bring encouragement, accountability, and useful ideas.

Remember, making moderate, incremental modifications to your eating patterns is more sustainable than dramatic limitations. Aim for long-term lifestyle changes rather than short-term diets to maintain a healthy relationship with food and accomplish your objectives.

Controlling portion sizes plays a significant part in keeping a healthy diet. By adopting portion controls, you may limit your calorie consumption, establish a balanced nutritional intake, and promote weight management.

It's crucial to be attentive to your body's hunger and fullness signals, use smaller plates and bowls, and plan and prepare your meals in advance. Incorporating protein and fiber-rich meals, keeping hydrated, and preventing junk food and sugary snacks are further healthy approaches.

Remember to be mindful of emotional eating triggers and seek assistance and accountability when required. By following these portion management tactics and creating a mindful attitude to eating, you can take responsibility for your dietary habits, improve general well-being, and live a balanced and fulfilling lifestyle.

In conclusion, adopting a fulfilled and diversified diet may have various advantages for your general well-being and pleasure of food. By concentrating on satisfaction, you emphasize picking meals that both fuel your body and please your taste senses, fostering a healthy connection with food. This technique provides for flexibility and diversity, guaranteeing that you may experience a broad range of tastes, textures, and cuisines.

A fulfilled and diversified diet promotes balance and moderation, rather than severe rules or limits.

It encourages you to listen to your body's signals, eat consciously, and make conscious decisions that promote your health and pleasure. This method may help eliminate feelings of deprivation, lower the likelihood of disordered eating, and develop a sustainable and long-term attitude to healthy eating.

By combining a range of nutrient-dense meals, such as fruits, vegetables, whole grains, lean proteins, and healthy fats, you may guarantee that your body obtains a broad assortment of necessary nutrients. This variety not only helps physical health but also adds to gastronomic delight and cuisine discovery.

A fulfilled and diversified diet also allows for the occasional splurge or exceptional pleasures, as long as they are enjoyed in moderation. This technique helps build a healthy relationship with food, where no items are off-limits, and guilt or shame connected with eating is reduced.

Furthermore, a satisfying and diversified diet develops a favorable mentality towards food and eating. It encourages you to enjoy the delights of food, participate in communal eating experiences, and discover new tastes and ingredients.

This may lead to a better feeling of happiness and fulfillment in your whole eating experience.

In summary, adopting a fulfilled and diverse diet gives a balanced and comprehensive approach to nutrition. By emphasizing satisfaction, variety, and moderation, you may build a pleasant and sustainable eating pattern that supports your overall well-being, fosters a healthy connection with food, and enables you to enjoy the joys of eating to the fullest.